THE LYME DISEASE COOKBOOK

Dr. Kimberly Carlos

Copyright © 2023 by Dr. Kimberly Carlos

All rights reserved. No part of this publication may be reproduced, distributed, or transmitted in any form or by any means, including photocopying, recording, or other electronic or mechanical methods, without the prior written permission of the publisher, except in the case of brief quotations embodied in critical reviews and certain other noncommercial uses permitted by copyright law.

TABLE OF CONTENT

INTRODUCTION

Once, in a quiet corner of a quaint countryside town, there lived a woman named Emily who faced a relentless battle with Lyme disease. The ailment had turned her vibrant life into a daily struggle, overshadowing her dreams and aspirations. Doctors had prescribed countless medications and treatments, yet relief remained elusive.

One day, while browsing the internet for alternative treatments, Emily stumbled upon a story of hope. It was about Sarah, a woman who had successfully overcome Lyme disease through the power of nutrition. Intrigued, Emily decided to give it a try, as she had nothing left to lose.

Emily embarked on a journey to transform her diet. She embraced a diet rich in organic fruits and vegetables, lean proteins, and whole grains. She eliminated processed foods, sugars, and gluten. Emily also incorporated immune-boosting supplements and herbal teas known for their antibacterial properties.

As weeks turned into months, Emily noticed subtle improvements. Her energy levels increased, and the relentless joint pain began to wane. The debilitating fatigue that had once confined her to her bed slowly lifted.

Emily's story of determination and dietary transformation spread through the Lyme disease support community, inspiring others to explore the healing potential of nutrition. She connected with a holistic health coach who guided her on this journey, providing emotional support and tailored meal plans.

Years passed, and Emily's Lyme disease symptoms became a distant memory. She returned to the activities she once loved: hiking through the lush woods, tending to her garden, and even taking up painting. Emily's remarkable recovery not only transformed her life but also ignited a beacon of hope for countless others who believed that healing could be found in the simplest of choices – the food they put on their plates.

Emily's story became a testament to the remarkable healing power of the right diet, a beacon of hope for all those who faced similar battles. Through her courage and resilience, she not only cured her Lyme disease but also inspired a community to embrace the healing potential of nourishing their bodies with the right nutrients.

CHAPTER ONE

Lyme disease: Types, Causes and Symptoms

Lyme disease, also known as Lyme borreliosis, is a tick-borne illness caused by the bacterium Borrelia burgdorferi. It's one of the most common vector-borne diseases in the United States and Europe. Lyme disease presents a wide range of symptoms that can affect various body systems, and it often progresses through distinct stages.

Understanding its types, causes, and symptoms is crucial for early diagnosis and effective treatment.

Types of Lyme Disease

1. Early Localized Lyme Disease: In this initial stage, symptoms are often mild and localized around the site of the tick bite. Common symptoms include a red, circular rash (erythema migrans) and flu-like symptoms such as fatigue, fever, headache, and muscle and joint aches.

2. Early Disseminated Lyme Disease: If left untreated, Lyme disease can progress to this stage, typically occurring several weeks to months after the initial infection. Symptoms may include multiple rashes, joint pain, and neurological issues such as Bell's palsy (facial muscle weakness) and meningitis (inflammation of the membranes surrounding the brain).

3. Late Lyme Disease: This stage can develop months to years after infection if the disease remains untreated. Symptoms often involve severe joint pain and swelling, neurological abnormalities, and cardiac problems like heart palpitations and arrhythmias.

Causes of Lyme Disease

1. Bacterial Transmission: Lyme disease is primarily caused by the bacterium Borrelia burgdorferi. It is transmitted to humans through the bite of infected black-legged ticks, also known as deer ticks, in North America, and Ixodes ricinus or Ixodes persulcatus in Europe and Asia.

2. Tick Habitat: Ticks carrying the Borrelia bacterium typically inhabit wooded and grassy areas. When a tick bites an infected animal, it can acquire the bacteria, and if it later bites a human, it can transmit the bacteria, leading to Lyme disease.

Common Symptoms of Lyme Disease

1. Erythema Migrans: A circular, expanding rash with a central clearing, often described as resembling a "bull's-eye."

2. Flu-Like Symptoms: Fever, chills, fatigue, headache, and muscle and joint aches can mimic the flu.

3. Neurological Symptoms: This may include numbness or tingling in extremities, memory problems, and difficulty concentrating.

4. Joint Pain: Lyme disease can cause intermittent or persistent joint pain, often affecting the knees.

5. Cardiac Symptoms: In rare cases, Lyme disease can lead to heart palpitations, chest pain, and shortness of breath.

6. Facial Muscle Weakness: Bell's palsy, a temporary paralysis of facial muscles, can occur.

7. Eye Problems: Some individuals may experience inflammation of the eye tissues (conjunctivitis) or light sensitivity.

8. Late-Stage Symptoms: These can include severe joint swelling, cognitive impairment, and heart rhythm abnormalities.

Early diagnosis and treatment with antibiotics are crucial to prevent Lyme disease from progressing to more severe stages. Lyme disease can have long-term complications if left untreated, emphasizing the importance of awareness and prevention when spending time in tick-prone areas.

Following a Lyme disease Diet with Benefits

1. Consult a Healthcare Professional: Before making any significant dietary changes, consult with a healthcare provider or a registered dietitian who specializes in Lyme disease. They can provide personalized guidance based on your specific needs and medical history.

2. Focus on Anti-Inflammatory Foods:

- Incorporate plenty of fruits and vegetables, especially those rich in antioxidants like berries, leafy greens, and colorful vegetables. These can help reduce inflammation.
- Include healthy fats from sources like avocados, fatty

fish (e.g., salmon, mackerel), olive oil, and nuts. Omega-3 fatty acids found in fish can have anti-inflammatory properties.

- Use herbs and spices like turmeric, ginger, and garlic, which have natural anti-inflammatory effects.

3. Maintain a Balanced Diet:

- Include lean proteins such as poultry, lean cuts of meat, fish, and plant-based sources like beans, lentils, and tofu.
- Choose whole grains like brown rice, quinoa, and oats over refined grains.
- Limit or avoid processed foods, sugary snacks, and sugary beverages, as they can contribute to inflammation and weaken the immune system.

4. Support Your Immune System:

- Consume probiotic-rich foods like yogurt, kefir, sauerkraut, and kimchi to promote a healthy gut microbiome, which plays a vital role in immune function.
- Ensure you get enough vitamins and minerals, particularly vitamin C, vitamin D, zinc, and selenium,

which are essential for immune health.

5. Stay Hydrated: Drink plenty of water to help your body detoxify and maintain proper bodily functions.

6. Be Mindful of Food Sensitivities: Some individuals with Lyme disease may have food sensitivities or allergies that exacerbate their symptoms. Consider food sensitivity testing or an elimination diet to identify and eliminate trigger foods.

7. Adapt to Your Energy Levels: Lyme disease can cause fatigue, so listen to your body. If you have low energy, focus on smaller, more frequent meals to maintain your nutrient intake.

8. Avoid Alcohol and Caffeine: These substances can disrupt sleep and exacerbate symptoms in some individuals.

9. Manage Stress: Chronic stress can worsen Lyme disease symptoms. Practice stress-reduction techniques like meditation, yoga, and deep breathing exercises.

10. Stay Hydrated: Drink plenty of water to help your body detoxify and maintain proper bodily functions.

11. Monitor Your Symptoms: Keep a journal to track your diet and how it affects your symptoms. This can help you identify specific triggers and adjust your diet accordingly.

Benefits of a Lyme disease Diet

1. Reduced Inflammation: Chronic inflammation is often associated with Lyme disease symptoms. A diet rich in anti-inflammatory foods can help alleviate inflammation, leading to reduced pain and discomfort.

2. Enhanced Immune Function: Proper nutrition supports a robust immune system. A diet high in vitamins, minerals, and antioxidants can help your body fend off infections and support the healing process.

3. Improved Gut Health: A healthy gut microbiome is essential for immune function and overall well-being. Consuming probiotic-rich foods can promote a balanced gut flora, which is vital for digestion and immune health.

4. Increased Energy: Nutrient-dense foods can provide sustained energy levels, helping to combat the fatigue commonly associated with Lyme disease.

5. Better Nutrient Absorption: A well-balanced diet aids in the absorption of essential nutrients, ensuring that your body gets what it needs to function optimally.

6. Weight Management: Lyme disease treatment can sometimes lead to weight fluctuations. A healthy diet can support weight maintenance and promote a healthy body composition.

7. Enhanced Mental Well-being: Good nutrition can positively impact mood and cognitive function, helping to reduce brain fog and other neurological symptoms associated with Lyme disease.

8. Support for Antibiotic Treatment: If your healthcare provider prescribes antibiotics for Lyme disease, a nutrient-rich diet can complement the treatment by supporting your body's ability to heal and recover.

9. Minimized Food Sensitivities: Identifying and eliminating trigger foods through an elimination diet can help reduce symptoms related to food sensitivities, which can sometimes exacerbate Lyme disease symptoms.

CHAPTER TWO

14-Day Lyme Disease Diet Meal Plan

Day 1

- Breakfast: Greek yogurt with mixed berries and honey.

- Lunch: Grilled chicken salad with mixed greens, cherry tomatoes, cucumbers, and balsamic vinaigrette.

- Dinner: Baked salmon with quinoa and steamed broccoli.

Day 2

- Breakfast: Oatmeal topped with sliced bananas and a sprinkle of cinnamon.

- Lunch: Lentil soup and a side salad with mixed greens and avocado.

- Dinner: Roasted chicken with sweet potato and asparagus.

Day 3

- Breakfast: Scrambled eggs with spinach and tomatoes.

- Lunch: Turkey and vegetable stir-fry with brown rice.

- Dinner: Grilled shrimp with quinoa and roasted Brussels sprouts.

Day 4

- Breakfast: Smoothie with kale, pineapple, banana, Greek yogurt, and flaxseeds.
- Lunch: Spinach and feta stuffed chicken breast with a side of roasted carrots.
- Dinner: Baked cod with a quinoa and vegetable medley.

Day 5

- Breakfast: Cottage cheese with sliced peaches and a drizzle of honey.
- Lunch: Quinoa salad with chickpeas, cucumber, red onion, and a lemon-tahini dressing.
- Dinner: Grilled pork tenderloin with sautéed kale and quinoa.

Day 6

- Breakfast: Overnight oats with almond milk, chia seeds, and mixed berries.
- Lunch: Tomato basil soup and a mixed greens salad with grilled chicken.
- Dinner: Baked trout with brown rice and steamed broccoli.

Day 7

- Breakfast: Scrambled tofu with spinach, bell peppers, and turmeric.
- Lunch: Lentil and vegetable curry with brown rice.
- Dinner: Grilled vegetable and quinoa-stuffed bell peppers.

Day 8

- Breakfast: Whole-grain toast with avocado and poached eggs.
- Lunch: Turkey and vegetable chili with a side of mixed greens.
- Dinner: Baked chicken thighs with roasted sweet potatoes and green beans.

Day 9

- Breakfast: Greek yogurt parfait with granola, sliced strawberries, and a drizzle of honey.
- Lunch: Spinach and mushroom quiche with a side salad.
- Dinner: Grilled swordfish with quinoa and steamed asparagus.

Day 10

- Breakfast: Smoothie with spinach, banana, almond milk, and a scoop of protein powder.
- Lunch: Chickpea and vegetable stir-fry with brown rice.
- Dinner: Baked turkey meatballs with zucchini noodles and marinara sauce.

Day 11

- Breakfast: Oatmeal with sliced almonds, raisins, and a dollop of almond butter.
- Lunch: Tomato and basil bruschetta with a side of mixed greens.
- Dinner: Grilled flank steak with roasted sweet potato and broccoli.

Day 12

- Breakfast: Cottage cheese with sliced pears and a sprinkle of cinnamon.
- Lunch: Quinoa and black bean salad with corn, red onion, and lime vinaigrette.
- Dinner: Baked cod with a quinoa and vegetable medley.

Day 13

- Breakfast: Scrambled eggs with sautéed mushrooms and spinach.
- Lunch: Lentil soup and a side salad with mixed greens and avocado.
- Dinner: Grilled shrimp with quinoa and roasted Brussels sprouts.

Day 14

- Breakfast: Smoothie with kale, pineapple, banana, Greek yogurt, and flaxseeds.
- Lunch: Turkey and vegetable stir-fry with brown rice.
- Dinner: Grilled chicken with sweet potato and asparagus.

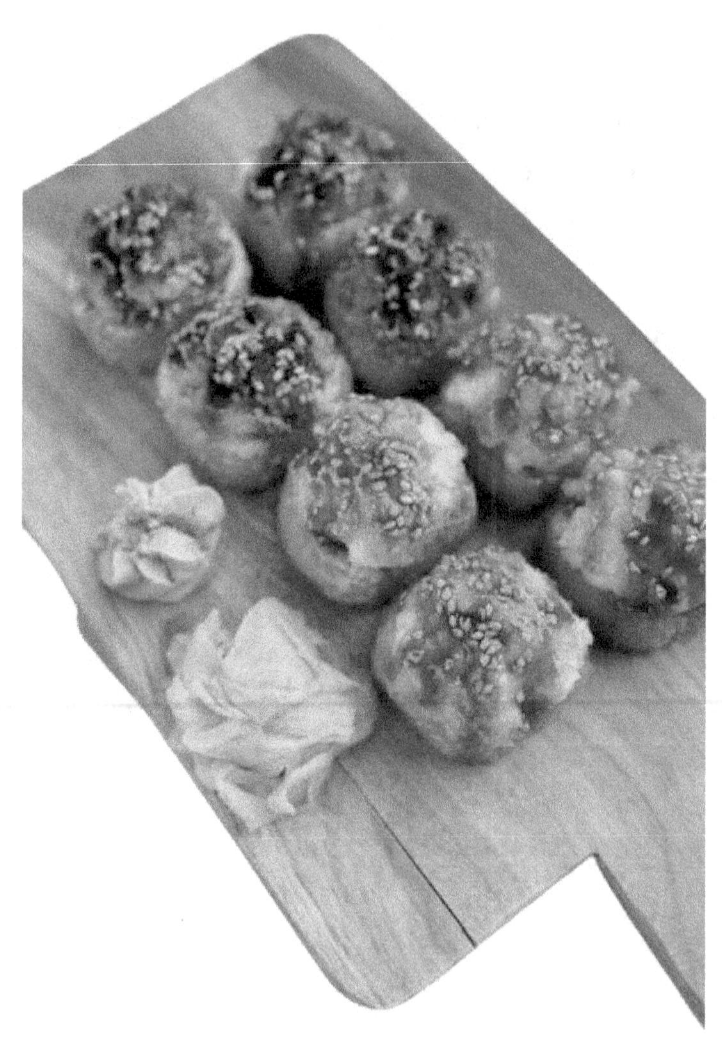

CHAPTER THREE

Lyme disease Diet Breakfast Recipes

1. Berry Smoothie Bowl

Ingredients:

- 1 cup mixed berries (strawberries, blueberries, raspberries)
- 1/2 cup Greek yogurt
- 1/4 cup rolled oats
- 1 tablespoon honey
- Sliced almonds and chia seeds for topping

Instructions:

1. Blend mixed berries, Greek yogurt, rolled oats, and honey until smooth.

2. Pour the mixture into a bowl.

3. Top with sliced almonds and chia seeds.

4. Enjoy!

Cooking Time: 5 minutes

2. Avocado and Poached Egg Toast

Ingredients:

- 1 slice whole-grain bread

- 1/2 ripe avocado

- 1 poached egg

- Salt and pepper to taste

- Red pepper flakes (optional)

Instructions:

1. Toast the whole-grain bread.

2. Mash the avocado and spread it on the toasted bread.

3. Place the poached egg on top.

4. Season with salt, pepper, and red pepper flakes if desired.

5. Enjoy!

Cooking Time: 10 minutes

3. Spinach and Mushroom Scrambled Tofu

Ingredients:

- 1/2 cup crumbled firm tofu

-   1 cup fresh spinach

-   1/2 cup sliced mushrooms

-   1/4 cup diced tomatoes

-   1/4 teaspoon turmeric

-   Salt and pepper to taste

Instructions:

1. In a non-stick skillet, sauté mushrooms until tender.

2. Add spinach and diced tomatoes; cook until wilted.

3. Stir in crumbled tofu and turmeric.

4. Season with salt and pepper.

5. Cook until heated through.

6. Enjoy!

Cooking Time: 15 minutes

4. Overnight Chia Pudding

Ingredients:

-   2 tablespoons chia seeds

-   1/2 cup almond milk

- 1/2 teaspoon vanilla extract

- 1 tablespoon honey

- Fresh berries for topping

Instructions:

1. Mix chia seeds, almond milk, vanilla extract, and honey in a jar.

2. Stir well and refrigerate overnight.

3. Top with fresh berries in the morning.

4. Enjoy!

Cooking Time: 5 minutes prep + overnight

5. Greek Yogurt Parfait

Ingredients:

- 1 cup Greek yogurt

- 1/4 cup granola

- 1/2 cup mixed berries

- 1 tablespoon honey

Instructions:

1. Layer Greek yogurt, granola, and mixed berries in a glass.

2. Drizzle honey over the top.

3. Enjoy!

Cooking Time: 5 minutes

6. Spinach and Feta Omelette

Ingredients:

-   2 eggs
-   Handful of fresh spinach
-   2 tablespoons crumbled feta cheese
-   Salt and pepper to taste

Instructions:

1. Whisk eggs in a bowl.

2. Heat a non-stick skillet and add spinach until wilted.

3. Pour eggs over spinach.

4. Sprinkle feta cheese on one half of the omelette.

5. Fold the omelette in half and cook until set.

6. Season with salt and pepper.

7. Enjoy!

Cooking Time: 10 minutes

7. Banana Walnut Oatmeal

Ingredients:

- 1/2 cup rolled oats
- 1 cup almond milk
- 1 ripe banana, mashed
- 2 tablespoons chopped walnuts
- 1 teaspoon honey

Instructions:

1. Combine rolled oats and almond milk in a saucepan.

2. Cook over medium heat until oats are soft and creamy.

3. Stir in mashed banana and chopped walnuts.

4. Drizzle with honey.

5. Enjoy!

Cooking Time: 10 minutes

8. Cottage Cheese with Berries

Ingredients:

- 1/2 cup cottage cheese

- 1/2 cup mixed berries

- 1 tablespoon honey

- Sliced almonds for topping

Instructions:

1. Mix cottage cheese and mixed berries in a bowl.

2. Drizzle with honey.

3. Top with sliced almonds.

4. Enjoy!

Cooking Time: 5 minutes

9. Almond Butter and Banana Toast

Ingredients:

- 1 slice whole-grain bread

- 2 tablespoons almond butter

- 1/2 banana, sliced

- A sprinkle of cinnamon

Instructions:

1. Toast the whole-grain bread.

2. Spread almond butter on the toast.

3. Arrange banana slices on top.

4. Sprinkle with cinnamon.

5. Enjoy!

Cooking Time: 5 minutes

10. Smoked Salmon and Avocado Wrap

Ingredients:

- 1 whole-grain wrap or tortilla
- 2 ounces smoked salmon
- 1/2 avocado, sliced
- Sliced cucumber and red onion
- Greek yogurt or cream cheese (optional)

Instructions:

1. Lay out the wrap.

2. Spread Greek yogurt or cream cheese (if desired).

3. Layer smoked salmon, avocado, cucumber, and red onion.

4. Roll up the wrap.

5. Enjoy!

Cooking Time: 10 minutes

Lyme disease Diet Lunch Recipes

1. Quinoa and Chickpea Salad

Ingredients:

- 1 cup cooked quinoa
- 1 cup canned chickpeas, drained and rinsed
- 1/2 cucumber, diced
- 1/2 red bell pepper, diced
- 1/4 cup fresh parsley, chopped
- Juice of 1 lemon
- 2 tablespoons olive oil
- Salt and pepper to taste

Instructions:

1. In a large bowl, combine quinoa, chickpeas, cucumber, red bell pepper, and parsley.

2. In a small bowl, whisk together lemon juice, olive oil, salt, and pepper.

3. Drizzle the dressing over the salad and toss to combine.

4. Enjoy!

Cooking Time: 15 minutes

2. Lentil and Vegetable Soup

Ingredients:

- 1 cup dried green or brown lentils, rinsed and drained
- 4 cups vegetable broth
- 1 onion, diced
- 2 carrots, diced
- 2 celery stalks, diced
- 2 cloves garlic, minced
- 1 teaspoon dried thyme
- Salt and pepper to taste

Instructions:

1. In a large pot, sauté onions, carrots, and celery until softened.

2. Add minced garlic and cook for another minute.

3. Stir in lentils, vegetable broth, thyme, salt, and pepper.

4. Bring to a boil, then reduce heat and simmer for 30-40 minutes, until lentils are tender.

5. Enjoy!

Cooking Time: 45 minutes

3. Spinach and Feta Stuffed Bell Peppers

Ingredients:

- 2 bell peppers, halved and seeds removed
- 2 cups fresh spinach
- 1/2 cup crumbled feta cheese
- 1 cup cooked quinoa
- 1/4 cup chopped sun-dried tomatoes
- 1/4 cup chopped fresh basil
- Salt and pepper to taste

Instructions:

1. Preheat your oven to 375°F (190°C).

2. In a bowl, mix spinach, feta cheese, quinoa, sun-dried tomatoes, basil, salt, and pepper.

3. Stuff the bell pepper halves with the mixture.

4. Place stuffed peppers in a baking dish, cover with foil, and bake for 30-35 minutes until peppers are tender.

5. Enjoy!

Cooking Time: 45 minutes

4. Tuna Salad Lettuce Wraps

Ingredients:

- 1 can (5 ounces) tuna in water, drained
- 2 tablespoons Greek yogurt
- 1 celery stalk, finely chopped
- 1/4 red onion, finely chopped
- 1 tablespoon fresh lemon juice
- Salt and pepper to taste
- Lettuce leaves for wrapping

Instructions:

1. In a bowl, combine tuna, Greek yogurt, celery, red onion, lemon juice, salt, and pepper.

2. Spoon the tuna salad onto lettuce leaves.

3. Wrap and enjoy!

Cooking Time: 10 minutes

5. Roasted Vegetable Quinoa Bowl

Ingredients:

- 1 cup cooked quinoa
- Assorted roasted vegetables (e.g., sweet potatoes, broccoli, bell peppers)
- 1/4 cup hummus
- Fresh herbs (e.g., parsley, cilantro) for garnish
- Olive oil for drizzling
- Salt and pepper to taste

Instructions:

1. Roast your choice of vegetables in the oven with olive oil, salt, and pepper until tender and slightly caramelized.

2. Arrange the roasted vegetables on top of the cooked quinoa.

3. Drizzle with hummus and garnish with fresh herbs.

4. Enjoy!

Cooking Time: 30 minutes

6. Chicken and Vegetable Stir-Fry

Ingredients:

- 1 boneless, skinless chicken breast, thinly sliced
- 2 cups mixed stir-fry vegetables (e.g., bell peppers, broccoli, snap peas)
- 2 cloves garlic, minced
- 2 tablespoons low-sodium soy sauce
- 1 tablespoon honey
- 1 tablespoon olive oil
- Cooked brown rice for serving

Instructions:

1. In a wok or large skillet, heat olive oil over medium-high heat.

2. Add chicken slices and stir-fry until cooked through. Remove from the pan.

3. In the same pan, add minced garlic and stir-fry vegetables. Cook until tender-crisp.

4. Return the cooked chicken to the pan.

5. In a small bowl, whisk together soy sauce and honey. Pour

over the chicken and vegetables.

6. Stir-fry for an additional 2 minutes.

7. Serve over brown rice.

8. Enjoy!

Cooking Time: 25 minutes

7. Smashed Avocado and Tomato Toast

Ingredients:

-   2 slices whole-grain bread
-   1 ripe avocado, mashed
-   1 large tomato, sliced
-   Fresh basil leaves for garnish
-   Salt and pepper to taste

Instructions:

1. Toast the whole-grain bread.

2. Spread mashed avocado on the toast.

3. Arrange tomato slices on top.

4. Garnish with fresh basil leaves and season with salt and pepper.

5. Enjoy!

Cooking Time: 10 minutes

8. Salmon and Quinoa Salad

Ingredients:

- 4 ounces baked or grilled salmon
- 1 cup cooked quinoa
- 1 cup mixed greens (e.g., spinach, arugula)
- 1/4 cup cherry tomatoes, halved
- 1/4 cup sliced cucumber
- Lemon-tahini dressing (1 tablespoon tahini, 1 tablespoon lemon juice, water to thin)
- Salt and pepper to taste

Instructions:

1. Place mixed greens on a plate.

2. Top with quinoa, cherry tomatoes, and cucumber.

3. Add flaked salmon.

4. Drizzle with lemon-tahini dressing.

5. Season with salt and pepper.

6. Enjoy!

Cooking Time: 15 minutes

9. Sweet Potato and Black Bean Salad

Ingredients:

- 1 large sweet potato, cubed and roasted
- 1 can (15 ounces) black beans, drained and rinsed
- 1/2 red onion, finely chopped
- 1 red bell pepper, diced
- Fresh cilantro leaves for garnish
- Olive oil and lime juice for dressing
- Salt and pepper to taste

Instructions:

1. Roast sweet potato cubes with olive oil, salt, and pepper until tender.

2. In a large bowl, combine roasted sweet potato, black beans, red onion, and red bell pepper.

3. Drizzle with olive oil and lime juice.

4. Garnish with fresh cilantro leaves.

5. Enjoy!

Cooking Time: 30 minutes

10. Turkey and Vegetable Wrap

Ingredients:

- 1 whole-grain wrap or tortilla
- 2-3 slices roasted turkey breast
- Sliced cucumber, red bell pepper, and avocado
- Leafy greens (e.g., spinach, lettuce)
- Greek yogurt or hummus (optional)

Instructions:

1. Lay out the wrap.

2. Layer roasted turkey, cucumber, red bell pepper, avocado, and leafy greens.

3. Add Greek yogurt or hummus (if desired).

4. Roll up the wrap.

5. Enjoy!

Cooking Time: 10 minutes

CHAPTER FOUR

Lyme disease Diet Dinner Recipes

1. Baked Salmon with Lemon and Dill

Ingredients:

- 2 salmon fillets
- 1 lemon, sliced
- Fresh dill
- Olive oil
- Salt and pepper to taste

Instructions:

1. Preheat your oven to 375°F (190°C).

2. Place salmon fillets on a baking sheet.

3. Drizzle with olive oil and season with salt and pepper.

4. Top with lemon slices and fresh dill.

5. Bake for 15-20 minutes until salmon flakes easily with a fork.

6. Enjoy!

Cooking Time: 20 minutes

2. Roasted Vegetable Quinoa Bowl

Ingredients:

- 1 cup cooked quinoa
- Assorted roasted vegetables (e.g., sweet potatoes, broccoli, bell peppers)
- 1/4 cup hummus
- Fresh herbs (e.g., parsley, cilantro) for garnish
- Olive oil for drizzling
- Salt and pepper to taste

Instructions:

1. Roast your choice of vegetables in the oven with olive oil, salt, and pepper until tender and slightly caramelized.

2. Arrange the roasted vegetables on top of the cooked quinoa.

3. Drizzle with hummus and garnish with fresh herbs.

4. Enjoy!

Cooking Time: 30 minutes

3. Grilled Chicken with Quinoa and Steamed Asparagus

Ingredients:

- 2 boneless, skinless chicken breasts
- 1 cup cooked quinoa
- 1 bunch asparagus, trimmed
- Olive oil
- Lemon juice
- Salt and pepper to taste

Instructions:

1. Preheat a grill or grill pan.

2. Brush chicken breasts with olive oil, season with salt and pepper, and grill until cooked through.

3. In a pot, steam asparagus until tender.

4. Serve grilled chicken over quinoa with steamed asparagus on the side.

5. Drizzle with lemon juice.

6. Enjoy!

Cooking Time: 30 minutes

4. Lentil and Vegetable Stir-Fry

Ingredients:

- 1 cup cooked green or brown lentils
- 2 cups mixed stir-fry vegetables (e.g., bell peppers, broccoli, snap peas)
- 2 cloves garlic, minced
- 2 tablespoons low-sodium soy sauce
- 1 tablespoon honey
- 1 tablespoon olive oil
- Cooked brown rice for serving

Instructions:

1. In a wok or large skillet, heat olive oil over medium-high heat.

2. Add minced garlic and stir-fry vegetables. Cook until tender-crisp.

3. Stir in cooked lentils.

4. In a small bowl, whisk together soy sauce and honey. Pour over the lentil and vegetable mixture.

5. Stir-fry for an additional 2 minutes.

6. Serve over brown rice.

7. Enjoy!

Cooking Time: 25 minutes

5. Mediterranean-Inspired Stuffed Bell Peppers

Ingredients:

- 4 bell peppers, tops removed and seeds removed
- 1 cup cooked quinoa
- 1 can (15 ounces) chickpeas, drained and rinsed
- 1/2 cup diced tomatoes
- 1/4 cup diced red onion
- 1/4 cup crumbled feta cheese
- Fresh basil leaves for garnish
- Olive oil for drizzling
- Salt and pepper to taste

Instructions:

1. Preheat your oven to 375°F (190°C).

2. In a bowl, mix cooked quinoa, chickpeas, diced tomatoes, red onion, feta cheese, salt, and pepper.

3. Stuff each bell pepper with the quinoa mixture.

4. Place stuffed peppers in a baking dish, cover with foil, and bake for 30-35 minutes until peppers are tender.

5. Garnish with fresh basil leaves and drizzle with olive oil.

6. Enjoy!

Cooking Time: 45 minutes

6. Spinach and Feta Stuffed Chicken Breast

Ingredients:

- 2 boneless, skinless chicken breasts
- 2 cups fresh spinach
- 1/2 cup crumbled feta cheese
- Salt and pepper to taste

Instructions:

1. Preheat your oven to 375°F (190°C).

2. In a skillet, wilt fresh spinach.

3. Cut a pocket into each chicken breast and stuff with wilted spinach and crumbled feta.

4. Season with salt and pepper.

5. Bake for 25-30 minutes until chicken is cooked through.

6. Enjoy!

Cooking Time: 35 minutes

7. Turkey and Vegetable Chili

Ingredients:

- 1 pound ground turkey
- 1 onion, diced
- 2 cloves garlic, minced
- 1 can (15 ounces) diced tomatoes
- 1 can (15 ounces) black beans, drained and rinsed
- 1 can (15 ounces) kidney beans, drained and rinsed
- 1 tablespoon chili powder
- Salt and pepper to taste

Instructions:

1. In a large pot, cook ground turkey until browned.

2. Add diced onion and minced garlic; cook until softened.

3. Stir in diced tomatoes, black beans, kidney beans, chili

powder, salt, and pepper.

4. Simmer for 20-25 minutes.

5. Enjoy!

Cooking Time: 35 minutes

8. Grilled Vegetable and Quinoa-Stuffed Portobello Mushrooms

Ingredients:

- 4 large portobello mushrooms, stems removed
- 1 cup cooked quinoa
- Assorted grilled vegetables (e.g., zucchini, red onion, bell peppers)
- Olive oil
- Balsamic glaze for drizzling
- Fresh basil leaves for garnish
- Salt and pepper to taste

Instructions:

1. Preheat a grill or grill pan.

2. Brush portobello mushrooms with olive oil and season with salt and pepper.

3. Grill mushrooms until tender, about 4-5 minutes per side.

4. In a bowl, mix cooked quinoa and grilled vegetables.

5. Fill each grilled mushroom with the quinoa and vegetable mixture.

6. Drizzle with balsamic glaze and garnish with fresh basil leaves.

7. Enjoy!

Cooking Time: 30 minutes

9. Shrimp and Vegetable Stir-Fry

Ingredients:

- 1 pound large shrimp, peeled and deveined
- 2 cups mixed stir-fry vegetables (e.g., broccoli, snow peas, carrots)

-   2 cloves garlic, minced

-   2 tablespoons low-sodium soy sauce

-   1 tablespoon honey

-   1 tablespoon olive oil

-   Cooked brown rice for serving

Instructions:

1. In a wok or large skillet, heat olive oil over medium-high heat.

2. Add minced garlic and stir-fry vegetables. Cook until tender-crisp.

3. Add shrimp and cook until pink and opaque.

4. In a small bowl, whisk together soy sauce and honey. Pour over the shrimp and vegetables.

5. Stir-fry for an additional 2 minutes.

6. Serve over brown rice.

7. Enjoy!

Cooking Time: 25 minutes

10. Baked Cod with Lemon and Herbs

Ingredients:

- 2 cod fillets
- Zest and juice of 1 lemon
- Fresh herbs (e.g., thyme, rosemary)
- Olive oil
- Salt and pepper to taste

Instructions:

1. Preheat your oven to 375°F (190°C).

2. Place cod fillets on a baking sheet.

3. Drizzle with olive oil and season with salt, pepper, lemon zest, and fresh herbs.

4. Squeeze lemon juice over the top.

5. Bake for 15-20 minutes until cod flakes easily with a fork.

6. Enjoy!

Cooking Time: 20 minutes

Lyme disease Diet Snacks Recipes

1. Greek Yogurt and Berry Parfait

Ingredients:

- 1 cup Greek yogurt

- Mixed berries (strawberries, blueberries, raspberries)

- Honey (optional)

- Chia seeds (optional)

Instructions:

1. In a glass or bowl, layer Greek yogurt and mixed berries.

2. Drizzle with honey and sprinkle with chia seeds if desired.

3. Enjoy!

Cooking Time: 5 minutes

2. Sliced Cucumber with Hummus

Ingredients:

- 1 cucumber, sliced

- Hummus for dipping

Instructions:

1. Slice the cucumber.

2. Serve with a side of hummus for dipping.

3. Enjoy!

Cooking Time: 5 minutes

3. Rice Cakes with Avocado

Ingredients:

- Rice cakes
- Ripe avocado, mashed
- Red pepper flakes (optional)
- Salt and pepper to taste

Instructions:

1. Spread mashed avocado on rice cakes.

2. Season with red pepper flakes, salt, and pepper if desired.

3. Enjoy!

Cooking Time: 5 minutes

4. Mixed Nuts and Dried Fruits

Ingredients:

- Assorted mixed nuts (almonds, walnuts, cashews)

- Dried fruits (apricots, raisins, cranberries)

Instructions:

1. Create your custom mix of mixed nuts and dried fruits.

2. Portion into small snack-sized bags for easy grab-and-go.

3. Enjoy!

Cooking Time: No cooking time

5. Carrot and Hummus Dippers

Ingredients:

- Baby carrots
- Hummus for dipping

Instructions:

1. Wash and prepare baby carrots.

2. Serve with a side of hummus for dipping.

3. Enjoy!

Cooking Time: 5 minutes

6. Apple Slices with Almond Butter

Ingredients:

-   Apple, sliced
-   Almond butter for dipping

Instructions:

1. Slice the apple.

2. Dip in almond butter.

3. Enjoy!

Cooking Time: 5 minutes

7. Guacamole and Veggie Sticks

Ingredients:

-   Assorted veggie sticks (e.g., bell peppers, celery, cucumber)
-   Guacamole for dipping

Instructions:

1. Wash and prepare assorted veggie sticks.

2. Serve with a side of guacamole for dipping.

3. Enjoy!

Cooking Time: 10 minutes

8. Chia Seed Pudding

Ingredients:

- 2 tablespoons chia seeds
- 1/2 cup almond milk (or milk of choice)
- Fresh berries for topping
- Honey (optional)

Instructions:

1. In a jar or container, mix chia seeds and almond milk.

2. Stir well and refrigerate overnight.

3. Top with fresh berries and drizzle with honey if desired.

4. Enjoy!

Cooking Time: 5 minutes prep + overnight

9. Cottage Cheese with Sliced Peaches

Ingredients:

- Cottage cheese
- Sliced peaches
- Cinnamon (optional)
- Honey (optional)

Instructions:

1. Spoon cottage cheese into a bowl.

2. Top with sliced peaches.

3. Sprinkle with cinnamon and drizzle with honey if desired.

4. Enjoy!

Cooking Time: 5 minutes

10. Baked Sweet Potato Fries

Ingredients:

- Sweet potatoes, cut into fries
- Olive oil
- Paprika (optional)
- Salt and pepper to taste

Instructions:

1. Preheat your oven to 425°F (220°C).

2. Toss sweet potato fries with olive oil, paprika, salt, and pepper.

3. Spread them out on a baking sheet.

4. Bake for 25-30 minutes until crispy.

5. Enjoy!

Cooking Time: 30 minutes

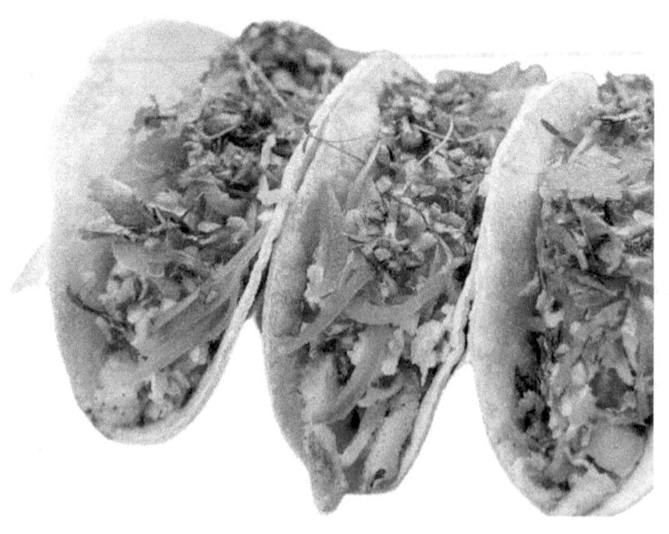

CONCLUSION

Planning a Lyme disease diet can play a crucial role in managing the symptoms and supporting the recovery of individuals affected by this complex condition. Lyme disease, caused by the Borrelia burgdorferi bacterium transmitted through tick bites, can lead to a range of debilitating symptoms, from joint pain and fatigue to neurological issues. While antibiotics remain the primary treatment prescribed by healthcare providers, a carefully crafted diet can complement medical interventions and enhance overall well-being. The foundation of a Lyme disease diet revolves around principles that include reducing inflammation, supporting the immune system, and promoting gut health. Anti-inflammatory foods like berries, fatty fish, and leafy greens can help mitigate the chronic inflammation often associated with Lyme disease. Additionally, immune-boosting nutrients such as vitamins C and D, zinc, and antioxidants can fortify the body's defenses against infections. A diet that prioritizes whole foods, lean proteins, and healthy fats can provide the necessary nutrients for recovery and healing. Incorporating probiotic-rich foods like yogurt and fermented vegetables can support a balanced gut microbiome, which is essential for immune function and overall health. It's important to tailor the Lyme disease diet to individual needs, taking into account any food sensitivities, allergies, or coexisting health conditions. Consulting with a healthcare professional or dietitian is recommended to create a personalized dietary plan that aligns with the individual's specific circumstances. While a Lyme disease diet can offer a range of benefits, including reduced inflammation, enhanced immune function, and increased energy, it should always complement medical treatment rather than replace it. Lyme disease is a complex condition that requires a multidisciplinary approach, including proper medical care, dietary considerations, and lifestyle modifications. In essence, a Lyme disease diet represents a proactive step towards managing this challenging condition. It empowers individuals to take control of their health, improve their overall well-being, and work in harmony with medical treatment to achieve the best possible outcome. By prioritizing nutrient-rich foods and making conscious dietary choices, individuals can embark on a journey towards better health and healing while living with Lyme disease.

www.ingramcontent.com/pod-product-compliance
Lightning Source LLC
Chambersburg PA
CBHW071105260726
48661CB00006B/2483